Clean Eating

Cookbook And Guide to Restore Your Body's Natural Balance and Eat Healthy

LELA GIBSON

CONTENTS

Introduction

I want to thank you and congratulate you for buying the book, *"Clean Eating."*

Nothing in life comes close to the value of good health. Taking your health for granted will only lead to a life of compromise. You will not be able to enjoy life or be happy, as you will be pressured into thinking about your health.

Good health is a measure of how much you care about yourself. The more you care for yourself, the healthier you become and the happier you remain.

But this is often easier said than done. Most of us tend to lead busy lives that prevent us from focusing on our health. We tend to go through stressful situations that impact our bodies negatively. Add today's lifestyle encourages the consumption of junk and processed foods that can cause health to backtrack.

The need of the hour is to, therefore, pick up a diet that is wholesome and capable of enhancing good health.

When we hear the word "diet" we are often reminded of salads and soups that do not taste good. However, not all diets ask you to settle for bland food that is stripped of flavor. In fact, you do not have to follow a fad diet to enhance health, as a clean diet will do the trick for you.

A clean diet refers to subjecting the body to clean foods. Clean foods are all natural and those that are free from chemicals and toxins. Staving off consumption of such foods can put your health on the right track.

To give you a head start, this book has been written to teach you the meaning and importance of clean eating. It provides you with simple recipes that can be adapted to enhance good health.

The book has been designed to facilitate easy reading and you will find it simple to navigate through the different chapters.

Thanks again for buying this book. I hope you enjoy it!

Chapter 1: Importance of Healthy Eating

Health is wealth and it is extremely important for people to take good care of themselves. It is especially important in this day and age, when people tend to load their bodies up with junk and processed foods. Before we explain why it is important to eat clean, we will first look at its meaning.

What is Clean Eating?

Clean eating refers to consuming foods that are natural and free from chemicals and preservatives. They include the likes of fresh fruits, vegetables, grains, legumes, pulses, oils etc. These are great for the body and will help you maintain good health.

Clean eating forbids the consumption of junk and processed foods. These are capable of negatively impacting your body. They promote the buildup of toxins that can, in turn, provoke illnesses. Clean eating subscribes to the principle that you should only consume those foods that are natural and which are good for the body.

Here are some of the rules that clean eating lays down.

- It is best to consume 6 smaller meals a day as compared to the regular 3 meals. Eating smaller meals can help the body to easily break down the foods and not feel burdened. But remember that it is the same 3 meals that will be split into 6 or 7 smaller meals, instead of 6 large meals.

- You meals should be made up of lean proteins and complex carbohydrates. Lean proteins help in the building of lean muscles. Lean muscles are tough to burn. You will be able to use up more energy while maintaining a lean body.

- You must incorporate a good dose of healthy fat in your diet. Not all fat is bad fat. Some fats help nourish the body and keep it strong. You must know how to incorporate the right fat in your diet.

- Clean eating stresses the consumption of 10 to 12 glasses of water per day. Water helps in flushing out all the toxins from the body. It also keeps you hydrated and enhances cell function.

- You have to eliminate all junk and processed foods from your diet. This includes the likes of take away, restaurant foods, packaged foods etc.

- You must refrain from indulging in bad habits that can adversely affect your health. These include smoking, drinking etc.

- Although not a part of the diet, it will be best to avoid stress as much as possible. Stress can upset your body and negatively impact your health.

Benefits Of Clean Eating

Weight loss

One of the biggest complaints these days is being overweight. Every other person in the world complains about weight gain. But nobody really puts in the effort to shed their weight and people invariably end up making the same food mistakes as always. The best thing to do to fix this situation is adopt a clean diet. The diet will not only help reduce your current weight but also prevent any additional weight from piling back on. But you will have to follow the diet closely in order to experience positive results. The foods consumed as per the diet are capable of melting your current fat with the consumption of liquids draining it away.

Digestion

Digestion is one of the most important activities of the body. It is only through proper digestion that your body will be able to separate the nutritional elements from the food you consume and direct it to all the right organs. Although most of us think we have a healthy digestive tract, it is often not the case. It might look as though your digestive system is functioning optimally but there will be a few issues to tackle. Shifting to clean eating can help solve these issues to a large extent. The diet will promote liver and gut health, both of which are important to maintain a healthy digestive tract.

Illness

Many people fail to understand that illnesses tend to build up over time. The food choices you make, the levels of stress you experience etc. all have a bearing on your body's upkeep. If you stick to bad habits for too long then you are bound to suffer the consequences. The diseases might not show up immediately but will impact your health negatively in the long run. By switching over to clean eating, you will be able to stave off the majority of illnesses. These can include the likes of certain types of cancers, cardiovascular illnesses and brain disease. Clean eating also helps in controlling diabetes to a large extent. But you will have to carry on with the practice long enough to see these positive results.

Immunity

It is vital for your body to have proper immunity. Immunity helps in staving off the onset of illnesses. You will be able to lead a better life if you prepare your body to limit illnesses. Right from a common cold to digestive problems, it is vital to keep illness at bay if you are able to. Clean eating helps in this regard and keeps common problems from arising too often.

Brain health

Brain health is just as important as physical health. It is extremely important for people to stave off the onset of depression and anxiety. These mostly come about if an individual makes wrongful food choices and or leads a sedentary lifestyle. It will be important to address both in order to experience positive benefits. Consuming a clean diet helps in increasing the dopamine content in the brain. This helps in keeping stress and anxiety at bay. It also increases serotonin, which aids in keeping the mind alert and active. Brain health, in fact, can have a direct bearing on physical health. Your body will be able to burn away more fat if your mind focuses on this.

Hair and skin

The clean diet helps in enhancing both hair and skin health. The consumption of fresh fruits and proteins helps in strengthening the hair follicles and gives your hair a unique shine. Fresh vegetables and elements such as vitamin E aid in enhancing skin health. They increase the collagen content thereby making skin more elastic. You will feel youthful and develop a unique glow. You will also be able to fight away wrinkles to a greater extent. Consuming the right type of foods can reverse your skin's age and leave you feeling confident.

Nail and teeth health

The clean diet has a positive impact on nails and teeth. Shiny nails and bright teeth can make a person look attractive. One of the best ways to enhance this is by following a clean diet. The abundance of omega 3 fatty acids in the diet helps in strengthening nails and teeth. The diet also promotes the consumption of foods that are rich in vitamins C and E that aid in maintaining nail health. You will have less complaints as you age and be in a position to maintain good oral health.

Adopting the clean diet can help you enhance productivity. You will be able to work better and get more out of your work life. The diet promotes the consumption of foods such as whole grains, fresh fruits and vegetables. These aim at increasing the level of dopamine in your brain, which is linked to productivity. They also decrease the cortisol level thereby enhancing brain function.

Better sleep

Sleep is one of the most important activities in life and yet many people fail to understand its importance. When you sleep, your body repairs itself from the inside. Defaulting on sleep will only lead to health issues. Many distractions tend to prevent people from falling asleep at night. The food they consume also has a big impact and can cause people to suffer from insomnia. Consuming clean foods can solve this problem to a large extent. The foods promoted through clean eating help in enhancing sleep and increasing the urge to sleep more.

Chapter 2: Foods To Keep Systems Clean

Clean eating involves the consumption of foods that are free from chemicals and additives. It focuses on ingredients that are natural and capable of enhancing the body's functioning.

Here are the clean foods to incorporate into your diet.

Foods To Include

Fresh fruits

Eat fresh fruits on a daily basis. Fruits contain many types of vitamins and antioxidants. These are required to keep your body healthy and prevent the onset of illnesses. They also help in keeping you looking youthful. You must aim at filling 20% of your plate with fruits. You can consume bananas, mangos, apples, grapes, pomegranates, watermelon, muskmelon, avocados, cherries, strawberries, lychee etc. Look for fruits that are in season and consume them as much as you can.

Fresh vegetables

You must consume fresh vegetables on a daily basis. One good way of incorporating vegetables is by picking 5 differently colored ones per meal. Say for example you pick carrots, peas, cabbage, tomatoes and yellow bell peppers. Try not to overcook them as they can lose their nutritional content. A simple salad or smoothie will make for a refreshing way to incorporate vegetables. You can consume tomatoes, okras, cabbage, cauliflower, beans, carrots, beetroots etc.

Lean proteins

Lean proteins are those that are free from fats and provide your body with the right amount of healthy proteins. They enhance your body's muscle building capacity. These muscles are tougher to burn and remain in your body for longer. There are many sources of lean proteins including fish, lean chicken and turkey, lentils, chickpeas, mushrooms, etc. You have to incorporate these into your diet as much as possible. It will be ideal to fill 30% of your plate with proteins.

Carbohydrates

Carbohydrates are an essential part of your diet. They provide you with adequate energy and assist with carrying out day-to-day activities. You must aim at consuming carbohydrates that are easy to break down. Brown rice makes for a better option as compared to white rice and whole wheat is good for your body as compared to white flour. A good trick is to have your heaviest meal just before working out so that you can successfully burn away the excess carbs.

Fats

It is a myth that fats are bad for your body. There are both good and bad fats and you must aim at increasing the good ones and decreasing the bad ones. The good ones are generally full of omega 3 fatty acids. These are important for brain and heart health. They contain a chemical known as DHA that is required by the body to remain healthy. A good source of omega 3 fatty acids is fresh water fish and flax seeds. Bad fats can build around your organs and turn into visceral fat. You have to avoid these in order to enhance good health.

Supplements

You can consider consuming natural supplements to enhance your health. Some of them include the likes of Ashwagandha, Gingko Biloba and green tea. They will help in flushing out the toxins from your body while encouraging good health.

Food To Avoid

The clean eating diet asks for the elimination of certain types of foods that are bad for the body. They are as follows:

Junk foods

You have to avoid consuming junk foods as much as possible. These foods can cause your body to not function optimally. They include the likes of fast foods, fries, pizzas, burgers, deep fried foods etc. It might not be possible for you to completely eliminate them from your diet but you must aim at limiting them to just once or twice a month. You can also consider preparing healthier alternatives that will not be as imposing on your body.

Processed foods

You must also avoid processed foods. Processed foods are packaged foods that can contain preservatives and other chemicals. Right from chips to biscuits to cookies, to cakes and other such foods, you have to avoid them at all costs. Sodas are also prohibited as they can fill your body up with sugar.

Apart from these, you must try to avoid alcohol as much as possible. Smoking can also negatively impact you and you must kick the habit to cleanse out the toxins.

Chapter 3: Clean Eating Recipes

Breakfast Recipes

Veggie Deviled Eggs
Ingredients:

10 eggs

2 tablespoons cabbage, boiled

1 avocado

1 potato, boiled

5 tablespoons peas

2 teaspoons mustard paste

Salt to taste

Pepper to taste

Paprika to sprinkle

Method:

Add the eggs to boiling water and allow it to hard boil.

Meanwhile add the avocado to a bowl along with the potato, peas and cabbage and mix well.

Add the mustard, salt and pepper and mix until well combined.

Once the eggs are done, peel them and cut vertically.

Scoop out the yellow and add to the avocado mash.

Spoon the mix into the cavities and sprinkle the paprika on top.

Serve warm.

Muesli
Ingredients:

1 cup muesli of your choice

2 strawberries, chopped

1 banana, chopped

1 cup yogurt

2 tablespoons honey

1 tablespoon chia seeds

1 tablespoon sunflower seeds

Method:

Add the muesli to a bowl and add in the strawberries and banana.

Add the yogurt bowl along with the honey and mix well.

Add it to the muesli and mix well.

Add the toasted chia and sunflower seeds to it and mix well.

Chia Pudding

Ingredients:

1-2 tablespoons honey

1/2 teaspoon vanilla extract

1/2 cup chia seeds

2 cups almond milk, unsweetened

Almonds for topping

Fruits like figs, blueberries, peaches and plums for topping

Method:

Mix the honey, vanilla, chia seeds and almond milk in a bowl, until well incorporated.

Allow the mixture to thicken in the fridge for a few hours or overnight.

Once frozen, stir well or add in some water in case you find the pudding too thick.

You can serve topped with fresh fruit and almonds.

Note: You can make your own almond milk by soaking almonds in water for 4 hours, then rinse and blend to obtain the milk. The pudding stores in the fridge for 5 days.

Almond Zucchini Muffins
Ingredients

1 tablespoon ground cinnamon

¾ cup unsweetened raisins

1/3 cup ground flaxseeds

1 ¼ cups whole wheat pastry flour

½ teaspoon sea salt

1 teaspoon baking soda

¾ cup blanched almond flour

¼ cup coconut oil- melted

1 ¼ cups finely shredded zucchini

1/2 cup pure maple syrup

2 teaspoons baking powder

Method

Preheat the oven to 350 degrees F and use 10 muffin fillers to line a muffin tray. Fill the empty slots up to halfway with some warm water.

Combine the almond flour, cinnamon, baking soda, pastry flour, flaxseeds, baking powder and salt in a medium bowl.

In another large bowl whisk together the maple syrup, ½ cup of water and coconut oil. Add in the dry ingredients to the wet ingredients and mix until combined.

Fold in the raisins and the zucchini gently into the mixture and add the batter to the ready liners.

Bake for about 20 to 25 minutes in the preheated oven or until a toothpick comes out clean after being inserted.

Allow the muffins to cool for 5 minutes in the tray and then transfer to wire rack to cool completely.

Wrap the muffins using plastic wrap and store them for 3 days at room temperature and for a month if frozen.

Banana & Chia Seed Toast

Ingredients

1 slice whole meal bread

1/2 medium banana, sliced

1 tablespoon sunbutter

1/2 teaspoon chia seeds

Method

Start by toasting the bread. Spread the sunbutter evenly over it.

Place the slices of banana on top of the sunbutter and then add the chia seeds as the final layer

Serve immediately and enjoy!

Main Meals

Chicken Wing Curry

Ingredients:

3 pounds chicken wings

1 large onion, chopped

1 jalapeno pepper, chopped

1 lemon, juiced and zested

2 cloves garlic, chopped

1 tablespoon coconut oil

1 cup chicken stock

Salt to taste

Pepper to taste

Cilantro to sprinkle

Method:

Add the onions to a pan along with the oil and sauté till brown.

Toss in the garlic and brown.

Add the peppers and sauté.

Tip in the chicken wings and brown it.

Add the lemon juice and mix.

Toss in the salt and pepper and mix.

Add the chicken stock and mix until well combined.

Sprinkle the cilantro leaves on top and serve.

Healthy Beef Stew
Ingredients:

1 large onion, chopped

2 teaspoons olive oil

1 large bell pepper, chopped

2 tablespoon jalapenos, chopped

4 garlic, chopped

2 teaspoons oregano

2 teaspoons coriander powder

2 teaspoons cumin powder

3 cups beef mince, cooked

4 cups spinach leaves

1 cup tomatoes, chopped

5 cups beef stock

1 lime, juiced and zested

Salt to taste

Pepper to taste

Parsley to sprinkle

Method:

Add the oil to a pan and toss in the onions and garlic.

Allow them to brown before adding in the bell peppers and sauté.

Add the oregano, coriander, and cumin and mix until combined.

Add the tomatoes, salt and pepper and mix well.

Add in the beef and beef stock and mix until well combined.

Cover and bring to a boil.

Once it does, add in the lemon juice and mix.

Toss in the spinach leaves and allow them to wilt.

Switch off the heat and sprinkle the parsley leaves.

Serve hot.

Easy Flat Bread
Ingredients:

1 cup wheat flour

Water to knead

Salt to taste

1 large carrot, grated

2 tablespoons vegetable oil

Method:

Add the flour to a bowl along with the salt and carrots and mix.

Add in a little water to make a firm dough.

Meanwhile, place a griddle on heat to warm up.

Allow the dough to rise for 5 minutes.

Make small balls out of it and roll it into circles.

Add a little oil to the pan and place one circle at a time to roast.

Flip once done.

Serve hot with your favorite stew.

Chickpea and Quinoa Bowl
Ingredients

½ cup cucumber slices

¼ avocado- diced

Pinch of ground pepper

⅓ cup canned chickpeas- rinsed and drained

Pinch of salt

½ cup halved cherry tomatoes

1 cup cooked quinoa

3 tablespoons hummus

1 tablespoon lemon juice

1 tablespoon roasted red pepper, finely chopped

1 tablespoon water

1 teaspoon chopped parsley (optional)

Method

Arrange the chickpeas, quinoa, tomatoes, avocado and cucumbers in a large bowl.

In another bowl, stir together the roasted red peppers, water, lemon juice and hummus.

Slowly add in more water to achieve desired dressing consistency. Season with some pepper, salt and parsley and stir well.

Serve together with the quinoa.

Lemon Rosemary Chicken & Potatoes
Ingredients

2 cloves garlic, minced

1½ teaspoons sea salt

3 cups baby red potatoes, quartered

3 tablespoons olive oil, divided

4 boneless, skinless chicken breasts

1 tablespoon fresh thyme, chopped

1 pound fresh green beans

Zest of 1 lemon

1 tablespoon lemon juice

1 teaspoon black pepper

1 tablespoon fresh rosemary, chopped

Method

Preheat the oven to 400 degrees F.

Whisk together lemon juice, garlic, thyme, pepper, 2 tablespoons of olive oil, zest, rosemary and salt.

In another bowl, toss the potatoes with some olive oil and season with pepper and salt.

Lightly spray a large baking sheet with oil and arrange the potatoes, green beans and chicken breasts.

Drizzle the mixture of herbs and oil over the ingredients using your hands or a brush making sure everything is coated nicely and evenly.

Put the pan into the oven and bake for about 25 to 30 minutes (it will really depend on the size of your breasts).

When done, the green beans should be nicely crisp, the chicken should have an internal temperature of around 165 degrees F and the potatoes tender.

Turn your broiler on for crispier potatoes.

Serve and dig in!

Barley-Stuffed Poblanos
Ingredients

3 slices reduced fat Monterey Jack cheese, halved

1 1/2 cups barley, soaked and drained

1 1/8 teaspoons chili powder, divided

1 (28-ounce) can crushed, whole peeled tomatoes,

6 poblano peppers

1 large onion, diced

1 bunch kale, leaves chopped, thick stems removed,

3 garlic cloves, minced

1/4 teaspoon kosher salt

2 ounces grated reduced-fat white cheddar

1/2 cup crumbled and pasteurized queso fresco

3 tablespoons olive oil, divided

Method

Add one tablespoon of oil to a large sauce pan and switch on the heat to medium high.

Add the onion and cook for 5-7 minutes, until soft. Add the barley and 3¾ cups of water and cook for about half an hour, until the barley becomes tender.

Stir the kale and 1/8 teaspoon chili powder into the barley and cook until the kale wilts, and then add in the cheddar and stir.

Now add the garlic to a pot with oil and cook for three minutes. Add the tomatoes, the rest of the chili powder and salt and leave it to boil. Reduce the heat and simmer, stir sporadically until the sauce becomes thick; this should take 30 or so minutes. Reduce the heat to low and cover.

Place the rack at the center and preheat the broiler. Slice off the stems from the peppers to create a wide hole for the stuffing. Reserve the stems. Remove the seeds and membranes carefully using a little knife.

Stuff the peppers tightly with the barley mixture and put back the stem ends to the top of the peppers.

Place the peppers in a broiler-proof baking dish and broil until the peppers become soft and charred, for about twenty minutes (don't forget to turn once halfway through).

Add the tomato sauce around the peppers and cover each one of them with half a slice of Monterey Jack. Now broil for 1-2 minutes, until the cheese melts.

Transfer the peppers to a plate and top each one of them with a tablespoon of the sauce.

Enjoy!

Onion Soup with Parmesan Croutes
Ingredients

For the Soup

2 teaspoons kosher salt

6 tablespoons extra-virgin olive oil, divided

2½ cups shallots, sliced

8 cups red onions, halved and sliced

1 teaspoon ground pepper

2 tablespoons chopped fresh thyme

10 cups beef broth (low-sodium)

8 cups leeks, halved and sliced (pale green and white parts only)

1 bunch scallions, thinly sliced

16 cups sweet onions, halved and thinly sliced

½ cup finely chopped fresh parsley

⅔ cup cognac or dry sherry

8 cloves garlic, sliced

For the Parmesan Croutes

2 tablespoons extra virgin olive oil

12 slices whole grain baguette, about ½ inch thick

1 cup grated Parmesan cheese

Method

Let's start with the soup.

Add three tablespoons of the oil to a large stockpot and heat over medium heat.

Add in the leeks and stir occasionally to ensure they are well cooked (softened but not browned for about 8-10 minutes).

Add the scallions, garlic and shallots then let them cook, still stirring for a minute.

Add the red onions, pepper, salt, sweet onions and the rest of the oil. Stir well to mix. Cook while stirring from time to time until the onions reduce by half, become very juicy, for about 45 minutes.

Add thyme, parsley and cook, while stirring from time to time until you notice the mixture turning deep brown, between 35 and 45 minutes or more.

Increase the heat to high and add sherry or cognac then cook for one minute, scrape up the browned bits for a minute then add broth. Now cover and leave it to boil. Reduce the heat, cover partially and let it simmer for 15 minutes

Meanwhile, let's prepare the croutes.

Place the oven rack in the upper third and preheat the boiler on low heat. Lay the slices of baguette on a baking sheet and brush one side with oil. Broil until they turn golden brown for about 4- 6 minutes.

Turn over the slices and top each one of them with a generous tablespoon of Parmesan. Broil until the cheese melts, for about 4 to 6 minutes. Top the soup with croutes and serve.

Store the soup for up to three days or freeze (could go for up to three months).

Tomato & caper linguine

Ingredients

400g dried linguine

350g tomato passata

1 lemon

Olive oil

5 tablespoons baby capers

Parmesan cheese

Method

Bring to a boil, salted water; add the linguine and let it cook (see the packet instructions).

Add some oil to a medium saucepan, place it over medium heat then add the rinsed capers and tomato passata and then grate in half of the lemon zest finely.

Give it about 5- 7 minutes to simmer before and seasoning with black pepper and sea salt to taste.

When the linguine is firm to the bite (not too soft), drain and then toss it with the sauce to coat it.

Grate it over some parmesan and if desired, some extra lemon zest and serve.

Snacks and Desserts

Fish Sticks

Ingredients:

2 pounds cod or tilapia cut into strips

2 cups almond flour

4 large eggs

Salt to taste

Pepper to taste

5 tablespoons coconut oil

Method:

Add the flour and salt in a bowl and mix.

Add the eggs to a bowl and whisk.

Place a griddle on the stove to heat up.

Dip the fish in the eggs followed by the flour and place on the hot griddle.

Pour some oil on top and brush it over.

Flip the fish and repeat the same.

Fry on both sides until completely crispy.

You can add it to a preheated 350 oven for 10 minutes to further crisp it up.

Serve hot.

Peanut Butter Cookies

Ingredients:

2 eggs

2 cups peanut butter (preferably homemade)

2/3 cup brown sugar

1 teaspoon baking soda

½ cup unsweetened cocoa powder

1 teaspoon vanilla extract

2 cups peanut butter chips

Method:

Break the eggs into a bowl and whisk until light and fluffy.

Add in the peanut butter along with the sugar, soda, cocoa powder and vanilla and mix until well combined.

Add peanut butter chips and fold gently until smooth.

Grease a baking tray or add a paper to the bottom.

Add 1 tablespoon of the mixture on top and spread a little.

Place in a preheated 300 F oven for 15 minutes or until the cookies are done.

Allow it to cool down for 10 minutes and serve.

Healthy Chocolate-Peanut Butter Bars

Ingredients:

For the crust:

3 tablespoons melted unsalted butter

24 chocolate wafer cookies

4 ounces semisweet, melted chocolate morsels

Cooking spray

For the filing

4 ounces reduced-fat cream cheese

1/2 cup 2% Greek yogurt

1/2 cup creamy all-natural peanut butter

2/3 cup confectioners' sugar

For the topping

Kosher salt

1/4 cup chopped roasted unsalted peanuts

Method:

Let's begin with the crust.

Get an 8-inch square pan and line it with foil (which should also overhang on two sides) and coat with cooking spray lightly.

Add the cookies into a food processor and process until fine and then add the melted butter and process once more up until the crumbs become coated with the butter.

Now add the melted chocolate, process until the mixture has the texture of wet sand. Press the mixture into the prepared pan using an offset spatula then cover and refrigerate as you prepare the filing. Clean the food processor bowl out.

The next step is preparing the filing and topping.

Add the peanut butter, cream cheese, sugar and yoghurt to the food processor's bowl and process until combined and smooth.

Pour the mixture on the crust and use a spatula to smooth it. Place the peanuts on top and sprinkle a ¼ teaspoon of salt. Cover it and leave in the fridge until set a bit looser than the cream cheese, roughly four hours up to overnight.

To loosen it, run a knife around the edges and lift it out using the foil handles. You can slice it into 12 bars but make sure you serve chilled.

Natural Flan

Ingredients:

3 cups coconut milk

5 large egg, beaten

2 teaspoons pure vanilla extract

2 tablespoons honey

2 tablespoons honey to caramelize

1 teaspoon lemon juice

1 tablespoon water

Method:

Add the coconut milk, eggs, honey and vanilla to a blender and mix until well combined.

Add the water, lemon juice and honey to a saucepan and allow it to caramelize.

Add it to a glass-baking dish and swirl around to coat the bottom.

Place this in a bigger tray with water in it.

Add the honey mixture to the dish.

Place in a preheated 350 F oven and bake for 15 minutes.

Allow it to cool down before serving.

Pecan Hotcakes with Berries

Ingredients:

1/4 teaspoon pure liquid stevia

1/2 teaspoon baking soda

1/2 teaspoon cinnamon, ground

2 teaspoons pure vanilla extract

4 whole eggs

8 ounce raw pecan pieces

Organic oil or grass-fed butter

Warmed frozen berries

Method:

1. Pulse the pecans in a food processor or blender to get a fine pecan meal.

2. Pour the pecan meal into a large mixing bowl and then whisk together stevia, baking soda, cinnamon, vanilla and eggs.

3. In a pan, warm some butter or oil and then ladle about 2 tablespoons of batter into the pan.

4. Cook the pancake until light and fluffy on both sides. Your hotcakes should fluff up when cooking.

5. In the microwave or pot, warm the frozen berries and then ladle them onto your hotcakes and serve.

Berry Bites
Ingredients

¾ cup plain Greek yogurt- low-fat

2 tablespoons coconut oil- melted

1 ½ cups fresh chopped strawberries and/or raspberries

¼ cup crushed almonds or almond meal

2 tablespoons honey

2 tablespoons coconut sugar, (add more for a sweeter Bite)

Method

Use parchment or silicone cupcake liners to line a 6-cup muffin tin or use a non stick muffin tin.

Stir together the coconut sugar, coconut oil and crushed almonds in a small bowl and spoon a small amount into each of the muffin cups.

Mix the honey and yogurt in a medium bowl and spoon 2 tablespoons into each muffin tin to cover the crust.

Top with some freshly cut berries and freeze for about 6 hours until firm.

To serve: peel out the silicone wrapper and let it sit at room temperature for about 8 to 10 minutes.

Enjoy!

Banoffee Parfaits

Ingredients

½ teaspoon vanilla extract (use vanilla paste for the speckled effect)

1 recipe of stove-top granola (recipe below) or 2/3 cup of granola of your choice

1 recipe of cooled date caramel (recipe below)

1 ½ cups plain yogurt (you can use a mixture of half Greek and half regular yogurt)

1 large- ripe banana

Method

Chop the banana into about ¼ inch coins.

Stir together the vanilla extract or paste with the yogurt.

Layer the ingredients in 3 small clean jars or glasses in the following order:

2 teaspoons of granola, a couple of banana coins, a teaspoon of date caramel, 2 tablespoons of the Greek yogurt and repeat for all jars or glasses. Once done, top the three jars with the remaining granola, caramel and banana.

Notes

Recipe for the date caramel:

Place chopped (and pitted) dates, ½ teaspoon of vanilla extract, 1/3 cup of milk and a pinch of salt into a blender and process until smooth.

Pour the mixture into a saucepan and heat over low flame as you stir for about 5 to 10 minutes or until reduced down and thickened: Let it cool.

Recipe for the stovetop granola:

Chop 3 tablespoons of almonds into rough small chunks and add to a small frying pan together with 1/2 cup of old fashioned oats and toast over medium heat for about 5 minutes.

Melt in 1 teaspoon of salted butter and stir in a heaped teaspoon of honey just until everything is evenly coated. Remove from the heat and set aside.

If you will be serving this later, place the sliced banana coins in some lemon juice to prevent discoloration.

To make the granola, you can use 3 tablespoons of any type of desired nuts or use 3 tablespoons of shredded coconut instead.

Variation for caramel apple pie parfaits: you can use ¾ cup of store bought or homemade applesauce mixed together with cinnamon to replace the banana coins.

Easy Salad Recipes

Traditional Egg Salad

Ingredients:

1/4 cup red onion, chopped finely

1/4 cup clean eating mayonnaise

8 eggs, hard boiled

Method:

1. Prepare the eggs by removing shells and then chop them into small pieces.

2. In a medium mixing bowl, put the chopped eggs, onion and mayo and combine well to blend. If necessary, add salt to taste.

Chicken Salad
Ingredients:

2 cups chicken, cooked and shred

1/4 cup walnuts, chopped

3 celery stalks, chopped

1 teaspoon rosemary

1 tablespoon vinegar

2 teaspoons olive oil

Salt to taste

Pepper to taste

Cilantro to sprinkle

Method:

Add the chicken to a bowl and toss in the walnuts.

Add the celery and rosemary and mix well.

Drizzle the vinegar, olive oil, salt and pepper and mix until well combined.

Serve with a sprinkling of fresh cilantro leaves on top.

Asian Vegetable Salad

Ingredients:

1/2 broccoli, chopped

1 large carrot, chopped

1 large cucumber, chopped

1 teaspoon sesame oil

1 teaspoon soya sauce

1 teaspoon White vinegar

1 tablespoon honey

1 tablespoon toasted sesame seeds

Parsley leaves to sprinkle

Method:

Add the broccoli, carrot, and cucumber to a bowl.

Add the sesame oil, soya sauce, vinegar, honey and salt to a bowl and mix until well combined.

Add it to the salad and toss until well combined.

Toss in the toasted sesame seeds and mix well.

Serve with a sprinkling of fresh parsley leaves on top.

Quinoa Salad
Ingredients:

2 cups quinoa, cooked

1 cup lima beans, cooked

½ cup mint leaves, chopped fresh cilantro, chopped

1 lemon, juiced and zested

1 tablespoon garlic powder

1 tablespoon honey

Salt to taste

Pepper to taste

Cilantro to sprinkle

Method:

Add the quinoa and beans to a bowl and mix.

Add in chopped mint leaves and lemon zest and mix until well combined.

Add the salt, pepper, lemon juice, garlic powder and honey to a bowl and mix well.

Pour it over the salad and mix until well combined.

Serve with a sprinkling of fresh cilantro leaves on top.

Chicken and Avocado Salad

Ingredients:

½ cup chicken, cooked and shred

1/4 cup carrots, chopped

1 large red onion, chopped

2 avocados, chopped

2 tablespoons balsamic vinegar

1 tablespoon olive oil

1 teaspoon mustard paste

1 teaspoon thyme leaves

Salt to taste

Pepper to taste

Parsley to sprinkle

Method:

Add the chicken to a bowl along with the carrots and onion and mix well.

Toss in the avocados and mix until well combined.

Add the vinegar and oil to a bowl along with the mustard, salt and pepper and mix until well combined.

Add this to the salad and mix well.

Sprinkle the thyme leaves and mix until well combined.

Serve with a sprinkling of fresh parsley leaves on top.

Egg and Tomato Salad

Ingredients:

2 eggs, boiled and chopped

1 zucchini, chopped

2 large tomatoes, chopped

1 onion, chopped

1 tablespoon vinegar

Salt to taste

Pepper to taste

Parsley to sprinkle

Method:

Cut the eggs into quarters and add to a bowl.

Add in the zucchini and tomatoes and mix well.

Toss in the onions and mix until well combined.

Add the vinegar, salt and pepper to a bowl and mix well.

Pour it over the salad and mix.

Serve with a sprinkling of fresh parsley leaves on top.

Spinach and Kale Salad

Ingredients:

1 cup spinach leaves, chopped

1 cup kale leaves, chopped

½ cup walnuts, chopped

1 avocado, chopped

Salt to taste

Pepper to taste

1 lemon, juiced and zested

Cilantro to sprinkle

Method:

Add the spinach and kale to hot water for 30 seconds.

Add to a bowl of cold water.

Remove and add to a bowl.

Toss in the walnuts and mix well.

Add the avocado and combine.

Add the lemon juice, salt and pepper and drizzle over the salad and mix.

Serve with a sprinkling of fresh cilantro leaves on top.

Fruit Salad

Ingredients:

1 red apple, chopped

1 green apple, chopped

1 orange, chopped

1/2 cup dried cranberries

1/2 cup chopped walnuts

1 cup plain yogurt

2 tablespoons honey

Method:

Add the apples and orange to a bowl and mix.

Toss in the cranberries and walnuts and mix.

Add the honey to the yogurt and mix until combined.

Pour it over the salad and mix well.

Serve cold.

Turkey Salad
Ingredients:

2 pounds turkey, cooked and shred

2 teaspoons garlic powder

2 teaspoons chili powder

2 teaspoons paprika

Salt to taste

Pepper to taste

1 avocado, chopped

½ cup corn

½ cup black beans

2 tablespoons salsa

1 tomato, chopped

1 onion, chopped

10 to 12 olives, chopped

Fresh cilantro to sprinkle

Method:

Add the turkey to a bowl along with the beans, corn and avocado and mix well.

Add the onion, tomato, corn and olives and mix well.

Add the garlic, paprika, chilli, salsa and salt to a bowl and mix well.

Pour this over the turkey and mix well.

Serve with a sprinkling of fresh cilantro leaves on top.

Couscous Salad
Ingredients:

1 large onion, chopped

1 cup spinach, chopped

1 cup garbanzo beans

1 cup olives, chopped

2 large tomatoes, chopped

2 avocados, chopped

1 tablespoon olive oil

2 cups couscous

1 tablespoon paprika

Salt to taste

3 cups water

Parsley to sprinkle

Method:

Add the couscous to a bowl along with the paprika, salt and water and allow it to swell up.

Add the onions, tomato, beans and olives to a bowl and mix well.

Toss in the avocados and mix well.

Once the couscous is done, add it to the salad and mix until well combined.

Serve with a sprinkling of fresh parsley leaves on top.

Smoked Turkey and Black Bean Salad
Ingredients:

2 cups cubed smoked turkey meat

4 cups field greens

1 teaspoon Dijon mustard

2 tablespoon cider vinegar

2 tablespoon olive oil

1 tablespoon minced garlic

¼ cup fresh cilantro: finely chopped

½ cup red onion, finely chopped

1 medium red bell pepper, chopped

1 cup shelled edamame, cooked and cooled

1 (14.9 oz.) can corn kernels, salt-free

1 (14.9 oz.) can black beans, rinsed and drained

Method:

Mix garlic, cilantro, onion, bell pepper, edamame, corn, beans and turkey in a bowl.

In a separate bowl, whisk together mustard, vinegar and the oil and then pour this mixture over the vegetables and turkey.

Toss to fully mix and then season using pepper and salt.

Once ready to serve, put equal amount of lettuce and then top with the vegetable and turkey mixture.

Beef Salad
Ingredients:

Sprinkle of oregano

1 chili, deseeded and sliced

2 handfuls lettuce

1 small cucumber, sliced

1 tablespoon crumbled feta

4 cups mushroom, sliced

2 cloves garlic, crushed

½ lemon, juiced

1 tablespoon olive oil

6 cherry tomatoes

300g Rump Steak, fully trimmed of fat

Method:

Drizzle the steak with a teaspoon of olive oil, small sprinkle of oregano and a clove of crushed garlic. Season with some salt and pepper too and set aside

Heat a griddle on high for about 5 minutes and then cook the steak on each side for about 3-4 minutes.

Put the salad ingredients in a bowl then sprinkle with sliced chili, squeeze of lemon, sprinkle of oregano, clove of crushed garlic and remaining olive oil. Use tongs to mix the ingredients thoroughly.

Remove the beef from heat and put it onto a plate. Allow it to rest while covered with foil, for 5 minutes.

Finally slice into strips before serving.

Artichoke and Asparagus Salad

Ingredients:

1 ounce shaved Parmesan cheese

1 pound medium asparagus, stems removed and cut into thirds

1 cup frozen green soybeans (edamame)

1 (14-ounce) can artichoke hearts, quartered

1/4 teaspoon pepper

1/4 teaspoon salt

1/2 teaspoon dried oregano

1 tablespoon lemon juice, fresh

2 tablespoons extra-virgin olive oil

1 garlic clove, peeled and halved lengthwise

Method:

Rub the insides of a salad bowl with garlic clove and then add in pepper, salt, oregano, lemon juice and oil. Whisk these until smooth.

Add in artichokes, toss the mixture slowly and allow to rest for some time.

Put the edamame into boiling salted water and cook for about 2 minutes.

Add in asparagus and cook the edamame and asparagus for 3 minutes. When crisp tender, rinse under cool water, drain and blot dry using a paper towel.

Add the edamame and asparagus mixture into the artichoke mixture, and then toss well to incorporate.

Finally distribute the salad among 4 individual plates. To serve, arrange shaved Parmesan over each salad.

Healthy Juices, Smoothies and Herbal Drinks

Spinach Juice

Ingredients:

2 celery stalks, chopped

½ cucumber, chopped

½ inch ginger, chopped

1 lemon, juiced

1 apple, chopped

2 cups spinach

Method:

Add the celery to a juicer and extract the juice.

Add cucumber and ginger and extract the juice.

Add the spinach, apple and lemon juice to a blender and whizz until smooth.

Combine it with the celery and cucumber juice and mix well.

Add in ice cubes and serve.

Cleansing Tonic
Ingredients:

1 teaspoon turmeric powder

2 carrots, chopped

1 apple, chopped

1 inch fresh ginger, chopped

1/4 cup orange juice

½ lemon, juiced

1 tablespoon honey

Method:

Add the carrots to a juicer and extract the juice.

Add the apple to the juicer and extract the juice.

Mix the two in a glass and add in the ginger.

Pour the orange juice and mix well.

Add in the lemon and honey and mix.

Serve cold.

Mixed Smoothie
Ingredients:

2 carrots, chopped

½ inch ginger, minced

1 green apple, chopped

2 stalks celery, chopped

½ cucumber, chopped

1 kiwi fruit, chopped

½ cup parsley, chopped

1 cup yogurt

1 tablespoon honey

Method:

Add the carrots to the blender along with the apple and ginger and whizz.

Add the celery and kiwi along with the cucumber and parsley and whizz.

Add the yogurt and honey and whizz until smooth.

Serve cold.

Beetroot Smoothie

Ingredients:

1 beetroot, chopped

2 carrots, chopped

3 stalks celery, chopped

½ lemon juice

½ inch ginger, chopped

1 cup yogurt

1 tablespoon honey

Method:

Add the carrots, beetroots, celery and ginger and lemon juice to a blender and whizz.

Add in the yogurt and honey and whizz until smooth.

Serve cold.

Orange and Strawberry Smoothie

Ingredients:

1 cup oranges, chopped

1 cup blueberries, chopped

1 cup orange juice

½ teaspoon salt

1 tablespoon honey

Mint leaves

Ice cubes

Method:

Add the oranges to a juicer and extract the juice.

Add the blueberries to the juicer and extract the juice.

Combine the two in a pitcher and well combine.

Add in the orange juice and mix until well combined.

Add the salt, honey and chopped mint leaves and use a muddler to crush the mint.

Add in ice cubes and stir.

Serve cold.

Digestive Drink
Ingredients:

1 cup Greek yogurt

1 cup buttermilk or regular yogurt

1 cardamom pod, seeds removed

1 small clove

½ teaspoon salt

1 tablespoon sugar

2 tablespoons mint leaves

2 tablespoons parsley leaves

Ice cubes

Method:

Add the yogurt and buttermilk to a blender along with the cardamom seeds, clove and blend until well combined.

Add in the salt and sugar and whizz until smooth.

Add in the mint leaves and ice cubes and whizz until smooth.

Serve with a sprinkling of parsley leaves on top.

Lemon and Mint Tea

Ingredients:

¼ cup lemon juice

1 cup mint leaves

1 teaspoon ginger, chopped

1 green tea bag

1 teaspoon black pepper

2 cups of water

1 tablespoon honey

Method:

Add the water to a pan and allow it to heat up.

Meanwhile, add the lemon juice, ginger, pepper and honey to a cup and mix well.

Add the tea bag to a cup and pour in the hot water.

Allow it to saturate.

Once done, add the tea to the juice and mix.

Serve hot.

Flower Tea
Ingredients:

½ cup rose petals, chopped

1 teaspoon black pepper

1 green tea bag

2 cups of water

1 tablespoon honey

Method:

Add the water to a pan and heat it up.

Add the petal and pepper to a glass along with the honey and mix.

Add the tea bag to a separate glass.

Pour one glass of water in the petals and another over the tea bag.

Allow them to steep for 10 minutes.

Mix the two together after straining the petals.

Serve hot.

Tomato Juice
Ingredients:

1 cup tomatoes, chopped

½ teaspoon ginger, chopped

½ teaspoon salt

1 tablespoon honey

1 cup mint leaves

Ice cubes

Method:

Add the tomatoes to the blender along with the ginger, salt, honey and mint leaves and whizz until smooth.

Add the ice cubes to a glass and pour the juice.

Serve cold.

Green Tea Spiced Tonic

Ingredients:

8 ounces purified water, near boiling

¼ teaspoon cinnamon

1/4 teaspoon turmeric

1 bag green tea

Method:

Into a tea cup, add in the teabag and the spices and then pour in the hot water.

Steep the tea and then remove the teabags. Stir to ensure that the spices are fully incorporated.

Super Juice
Ingredients:

Ice cubes

1 level teaspoon spirulina

1 ounce fresh Wheatgrass powder or Wheatgrass

½ avocados, ripe

½ cucumber, medium-sized

½ pineapple

2 apples

½ lime, peeled

Method:

Juice the apples, pineapple, lime and cucumber. Put the avocado in a blender and process until smooth then mix with the resultant juice.

Add the spirulina and wheatgrass and mix. Add in the ice cubes for a refreshing cold drink.

Purple Power Smoothie

Ingredients:

5 cashews

1 serving vanilla whey protein powder, unsweetened

1/4 cup pomegranate seeds

1/2 cup blueberries, fresh or frozen

1/2 cup raspberries, fresh or frozen

1/2 cup sweet cherries, pitted, fresh or frozen

1/2 cup water

Method:

Put the ingredients into a blender and process for around 60 seconds.

Serve and enjoy.

Kale Pear Smoothie
Ingredients:

5 raw cashews

1 serving vanilla whey protein, unsweetened

1 tablespoon lemon juice

1 cup pear

1 cup cucumber

1 cup kale

1 cup water

Method

Place all the ingredients in a blender.

Blend until smooth then serve.

I need your help...

Thank you again for buying this book!

I hope you had a good time reading it. The main aim of this book was to educate you on the basics of clean eating and what it can do for you.

You need not follow a fad diet to remain fit. You have to change your lifestyle as a whole and make better food choices. I hope you take the advice mentioned in this book seriously and put in the effort to enhance your health.

Finally, if you enjoyed this book, then I'd like to ask you for a favor, would you be kind enough to leave a review for this book on Amazon? It'd be greatly appreciated!

I want to reach as many people as I can with this book, and more reviews will help me accomplish that!

If you have any questions or problems, please contact us: hello@freedomdestination.com

Thank you and good luck!

Preview Of '20 Easy and Fast Diet Tips for Losing Weight'

Before we start learning about the strategies you can use to lose weight, let's start by highlighting some of the benefits that will come as a result of shedding those extra pounds just to give you extra motivation to want to do something NOW.

Why You Need To Lose Weight

Healthy weight loss has over one hundred benefits; these include emotional and physical benefits. I will dedicate this section to discussing the health benefits that many people (and weight loss/health books) do not pay enough attention to.

1: You Avoid Pre-Diabetes or Type 2 Diabetes

Pre-diabetes/high blood glucose is a condition that develops when the blood sugar levels in your blood move past normal ranges but not enough to qualify as diabetes. When your body stops consistently producing insulin sufficient to meet your body's needs, or the amount produced does not work properly, type 2 diabetes is likely to develop. Being pre-diabetic places you at a very high risk of developing type 2 diabetes.

Being obese or overweight is a proven leading risk factor for type 2 diabetes because carrying excess weight typically makes it hard for cells to respond to insulin, and since the additional fat acts as an insulating layer, it makes it more difficult for the sugar to enter the cells, which results in more circulating blood sugar levels.

Nonetheless, if you are already a pre-diabetic, you can prevent the progression to diabetes by shedding some weight (to reduce the insulating layer on cells so that they respond more to insulin) and trying to maintain a healthy weight.

2: You Keep Your Heart Healthy

When it comes to heart disease, some of the key risk factors are high cholesterol and high blood pressure. Research shows that:

1. Excessive accumulation of body fat makes your body release particular chemicals that occur naturally into the bloodstream, which increases blood pressure, and

2. Being overweight makes the liver produce too much amounts of Low density Lipoprotein (LDL) also called cholesterol. LDL tends to be sticky and gathers in the walls of blood vessels, which causes the narrowing of arteries, a condition called atherosclerosis, which increases your risk of strokes and heart attack.

When you lose weight, your blood pressure often reduces and the liver naturally reduces the amount of LDL it produces.

Royal Adelaide Hospital conducted a research on cardiovascular improvements with respect to a special weight loss program. Their results showed a decrease of cholesterol by 12%, a 10% decrease of LDL, a 5% decrease in diastolic blood pressure, and an 8% decrease in systolic blood pressure.

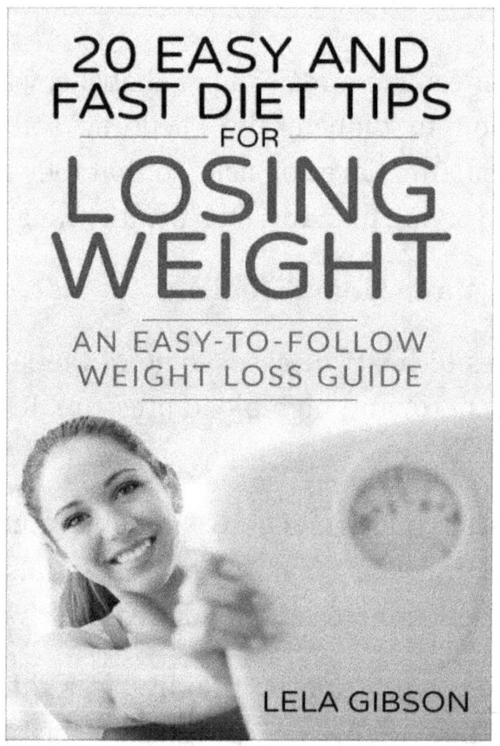

Check out the rest of 20 Easy and Fast Diet Tips for Losing Weight on Amazon., go to: **http://amzn.to/2kGyXvc**

Check Out My Other Books

Below you'll find one of my other popular books that are popular on Amazon and Kindle as well.

Alternatively, you can visit my author page on Amazon to see other work done by me.

Ketogenic Cookbook: Quick Low Calorie Ketogenic Crockpot Recipes with 7 Days Meal Plan

Freedom: How to Make Money Online and Become Financially Free by Creating Passive Income

Mediterranean Diet: Instant Pot Cookbook with Delicious Recipes

Alice the Superbug

Madison and Astrid's first magical journey

Intermittent Fasting: The Essential Beginners Guide for Women for Weight Loss

Chakra Healing: Chakra Healing and Karmic Awareness for Beginners

SEO 2017 for Growth: The Ultimate Guide to Learn Search Engine Optimization with Internet Marketing Tips

Psychology: How to Analyze People Using Human Psychological Techniques, Body Language Signals, Social Skills and Personality Types

Paleo Smoothies: Recipes to Energize and for Ultimate Health and Weight Loss

Belly Diet Smoothies: Delicious Smoothie Recipes to Flatten Your Belly, Improve Your Gut & Burn Fat

Keto Diet: Keto Diet Guide Cookbook for Beginners with Meal Plan and Simple, Delicious Recipes to Lose Weight and Look Good

Online Business from Scratch: The 9 Step Guide to Building a Profitable and Sustainable Online Business

Weight Loss: 20 Easy And Fast Diet Tips For Losing Weight - An Easy-To-Follow Weight Loss Guide

Ketogenic Cookbook: Ketogenic Cookbook for Beginners with 7 Days Meal Plan

Negative Calorie Diet: Cookbook & Guide Which Will Help You To Burn Body Fat, Lose Weight And Live Healthy

Negative Calorie Diet with Anti-Inflammatory Diet Guide

Make Money Online To Achieve Freedom

Negative Calorie Diet with Smart Fat Guide

Negative Calorie Diet & Clean Eating: Cookbook & Guide Which Will Help You To Burn Body Fat, Lose Weight And Live Healthy

Smart Fat: Cookbook with Fat Meals Which Help You to Lose Weight, Get Healthy and Improve Brain Function

Anti-Inflammatory Diet Guide: The Guide to Reduce Inflammation and Live a Healthy Life Without Pain

Essential Oils: The Young Living Book Guide of Natural Remedies for Beginners for Pets, For Dogs

Clean Eating: Cookbook and Guide to Restore Your Body's Natural Balance and Eat Healthy

Anti-Inflammatory Diet Guide: The Guide to Reduce Inflammation and Live a Healthy Life Without Pain

Dash Diet: Cookbook for Weight Loss with Action Plan and Easy Recipes

Air Fryer Cookbook: Quick, Healthy and Easy Low Carb Air Fryer Recipes

Psychology & Habits Of Highly Effective People Box Set

Leptin Resistance: Leptin Diet to Control Your Hormones, Get Permanent Weight Loss, Cure Obesity and Live Healthy

Negative Calorie Diet & Dash Diet Box Set

Negative Calorie Diet & Weight Loss Box Set

Habits of Highly Effective People: What Are the Habits of Successful People?

Slow Cooker: Cookbook with Slow Cooker Recipes

Weight Loss Cookbook: Meal Prep Cookbook for Weight Loss and Clean Eating

Weight Loss Cookbook: Mediterranean Diet for Lasting Weight Loss

Negative Calorie Diet & Dash Diet Box Set

Slow Cooker & Instant Pot Box Set

Children Books: Madison and Astrid's first magical journey & Alice the Superbug Box Set

Belly Diet: The Zero Belly Diet Step-By-Step Guide Which Helps You to Lose Your Belly and Enjoy Your Flat Belly

Weight Loss: 20 Easy and Fast Diet Tips for Losing Weight - An Easy-To-Follow Weight Loss Guide

Instant Pot: Instant Pot Pressure Cooker Cookbook with Easy and Healthy Recipes

Vegan Cookbook: Vegan Cookbook For Beginners, For Kids And For Teens For Diabetics With Pictures

Low Carb: Low Carb Diet Cookbook with Low Carb Keto Recipes for Batch Cooking

Ketogenic Cooking: Ketogenic Cooking With Your Instant Pot

Passive Income: Passive Income Tutorial with 7 Online Ideas to Generate Passive Income Streams for Beginners

Low Carb Diet: Low Carb Diet Recipes Cookbook for Beginners for Batch Cooking

Make Money from Home: How to Make Money Online and Escape the 9-5 Rat Race

Amazon Customer Service

Kindle Unlimited

Bonus: Subscribe To The FREE Cooking Ebook

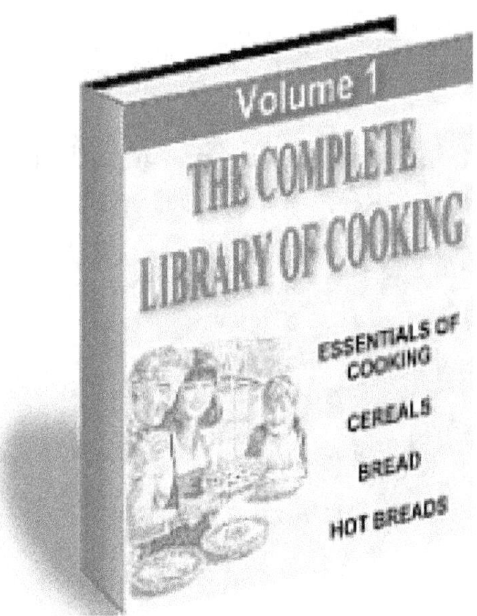

When you subscribe to Freedom Destination via email, you will get free access to an ebook. All you have to do is enter your email address to get instant access.

It is our hope that these volumes will help the you to acquire the knowledge needed to prepare daily meals that will contain the proper sustenance for each member of your family, teach you how to buy your food judiciously and prepare and serve it economically and appetizingly, and also instill in you such a love for COOKING that you will become enthusiastic about mastering and dignifying this art.

Here are the preview of what you'll get:

1. Essentials Of Cooking
2. Cereals

3. Bread

4. Hot Breads

To get instant access to these incredible ebook, go to: **http://bit.ly/2txvySs**

www.ingramcontent.com/pod-product-compliance
Lightning Source LLC
Chambersburg PA
CBHW070027260726
48658CB00002B/518